ALLEN PHOTOGRAPHIC GUIDES

ALL ABOUT WORMS

CONTENTS

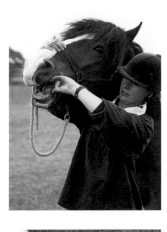

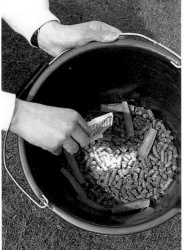

THE WORM PROBLEM

At the turn of the century, relatively little was known about equine parasites. They were controlled by dosing with one of a variety of substances including arsenic and turpentine or even by administering enemas of salt and water. Approaching the end of the century, there is far more knowledge about parasites and their effects on the horse, and there are more sophisticated drugs. As urban areas have spread, however, many owners have limited grazing for their horses which exacerbates most parasite problems. In the 1980s and early 1990s, there was a new difficulty, small redworms were shown to be developing resistance to Benzimidazole drugs at the same time as they were taking over from large redworms as the most troublesome of the horse parasites.

Worm parasites (often referred to as helminths) can adapt to different circum-stances and can build up to dangerous levels both inside the horse and in the environment. To be effective, our pasture management and use of drugs must take the current situation into account. No horse owner, however experienced, is exempt from keeping up to date.

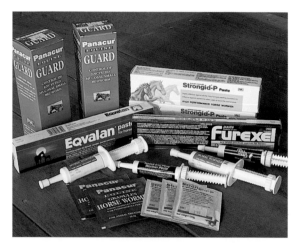

THE WORMS WE ARE UP AGAINST

NEMATODES These are cylindrical or 'round' worms

Small Redworm
Small strongyles, include 40 species of cyathostomes *Cyathostomum*
0.5–2.5 cm long. Life cycle 5–18 weeks. Can account for 90% of worm burden. Currently most common and potentially dangerous group of parasites. Some are now resistant to Benzimidazole drugs.

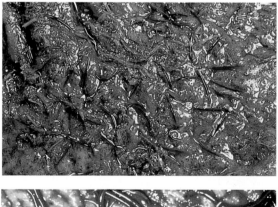

Large Redworm
Large strongyles. 56 species including *Strongylus vulgaris*
2–5 cm long. Life cycle 6–11 months. Red from sucking blood. Migrate through arteries. Not as common as they used to be.

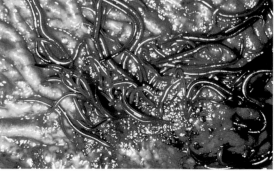

Large Roundworm

Ascarids

Parascaris equorum

30–50 cm long. Life cycle 10–12 weeks. Each day, one female can lay one million sticky eggs which are resistant to disinfectant and can survive for three years. Low level infection in most adult horses but can cause problems in animals under two years.

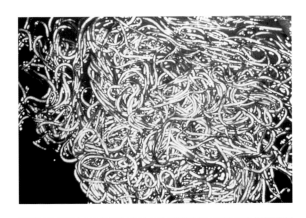

Pinworm

Seat worm

Oxyuris equi

Up to 10 cm long. Life cycle 4–5 months. Lays clumps of 50,000 eggs around rectum causing intense itching.

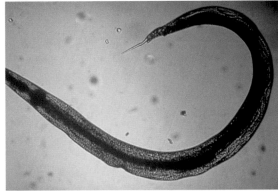

Threadworm

Strongyloides westerei

Less than 1 cm long. Life cycle 8–14 days. Lies dormant in adult horses but is transmitted in milk from mare to foal. Can also live freely in environment and can penetrate horse's skin. May cause severe disease in young horses but older animals are not affected.

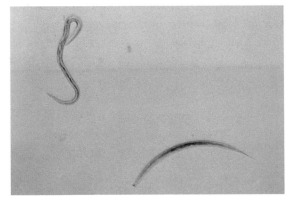

Lungworm

Dictyocaulus arnfieldi

Up to 8 cm long. Life cycle 2–4 months. Donkeys are preferred hosts. Will complete life cycle to egg-laying stage in donkeys and foals. If picked up by horses, may live in lungs without reproducing.

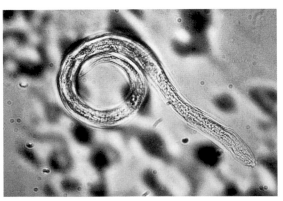

Stomach Hairworm

Trichostrongylus axei
0.5 cm long. Short life cycle of 3 weeks. Affects sheep, cattle and horses. Causes diarrhoea and weight loss.

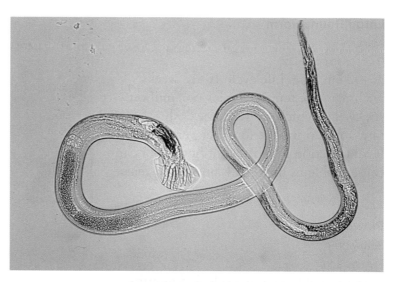

Stomach Worm

Habronena muscae,
H. microstoma
1–3.5 cm long. Indirect life cycle. Maggots pick up larvae from manure. When maggots mature to adult flies, larvae are deposited on horse when flies feed and are licked off by horse.

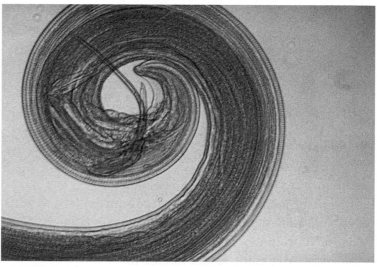

Neck Threadworm

Onchocerca cervicalis
5–30 cm long. Lives under the skin. Microfilariae, the embryonic larvae, are 0.25 mm long and are found in the skin tissue. Indirect life cycle of one month. Transmitted to horse via biting midges.

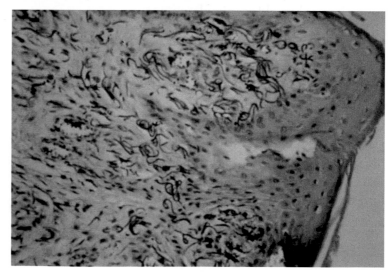

CESTODES (Flatworm)

Tapeworm

Anoplocephala perfoliata, A. magna
Up to 80 cm long. Indirect
life cycle of 3–5 months.
The intermediate hosts
are forage or oribatid mites
which survive on bedding
and pasture. Horse
consumes when grazing.

TREMATODES

(Flatworm with hooks and
suckers)

Liverfluke

Fasciola hepatica
Grey/brown. Indirect life
cycle of 3–4 months.
Common in mild, wet areas
like Ireland. A snail is the
intermediate host. Affects
cattle, sheep, horses and
donkeys. Only low burdens
usually found in the horse.
Causes anaemia and weight
loss. Not covered by routine
worming.

INSECTS

Bots

Gasterophilus: Several species
Maggot-like larvae of bot
flies, 2 cm long. Life cycle 1
year. Flies lay eggs on horse
from July to September.
Horse consumes eggs. Larvae
develop in stomach during
winter after migrating
through mouth and cheeks.
Passed out in the spring and
develop into flies.

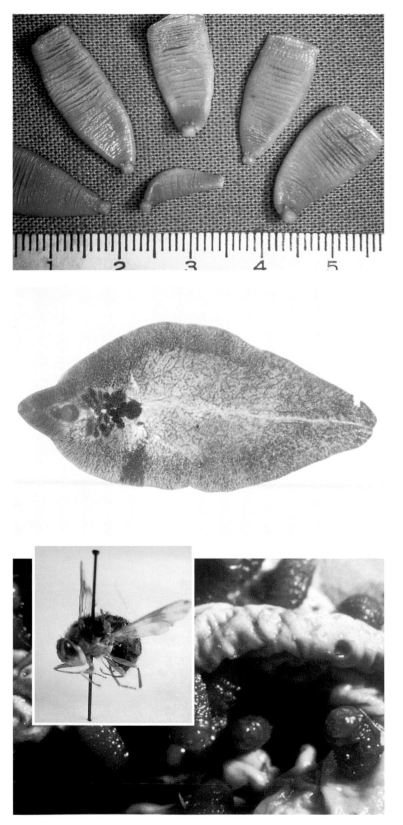

LIFE CYCLES

Most equine nematode parasites have a **direct life cycle**. There can be millions of eggs and larvae so the vicious circle needs to be broken at as many places as possible.

If another organism becomes an intermediate host by picking up larvae before transferring them to the horse, this creates an **indirect life cycle** (e.g. tapeworm).

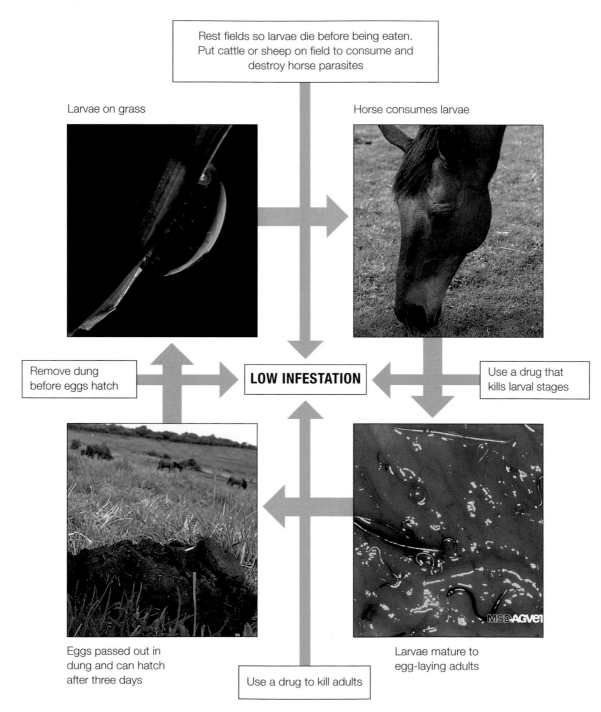

Rest fields so larvae die before being eaten. Put cattle or sheep on field to consume and destroy horse parasites

Larvae on grass

Horse consumes larvae

Remove dung before eggs hatch

LOW INFESTATION

Use a drug that kills larval stages

Eggs passed out in dung and can hatch after three days

Use a drug to kill adults

Larvae mature to egg-laying adults

Simultaneous life cycles Many species of parasite infest the horse at the same time. An ideal worming programme should include different drugs to kill all species.

Overlapping life cycles At any time, the horse may have many worms of different species at different stages of development. There will be larvae which have just been consumed, larvae migrating through the body or encysted in the wall of the intestine and adults in the intestine with eggs being continually passed in the dung.

In the chart below, each group of large redworm larvae ingested in a particular month is represented by a colour which indicates the life cycle stage the group has reached.

MONTH 1	MONTH 2	MONTH 3	MONTH 4	MONTH 5	MONTH 6
Ingested	Penetrate bowel	Migrate	Migrate	Return to bowel	Lay eggs
	Ingested	Penetrate bowel	Migrate	Migrate	Return to bowel
		Ingested	Penetrate bowel	Migrate	Migrate
			Ingested	Penetrate bowel	Migrate
				Ingested	Penetrate bowel
					Ingested

If the horse is wormed at the end of month 6 we can see what group of large redworm will remain in the horse after using different drugs.

Month 6 – drug administered
Ivermectin or a five-day course of Fenbendazole: most worms in all the groups will be destroyed.

Pyrantel or a routine dose of a Benzimidazole:

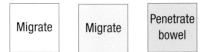

These three groups will be left in the horse's body, because the drugs are not effective against them. Therefore, there will be more egg-laying adults in the gut within a short time, which is why these drugs need to be used more frequently. It is important to remember that this chart is for only one species of large redworm. With tapeworm, for example, Ivermectin would be ineffective whereas a double dose of Pyrantel would be the treatment of choice.

Summary
- Life cycles must be broken at as many places as possible.
- Horses are infested with different species of worms at different stages of development at the same time.
- A combination of drugs is required to deal with the range of species and stages.

HOW SOMETHING SO SMALL KILLS SOMETHING SO BIG

Internal damage from parasites can cause serious disease which may be fatal, and at best it causes food to be wasted and prevents the horse from reaching its full potential. The donkey pictured here is suffering from a severe worm problem.

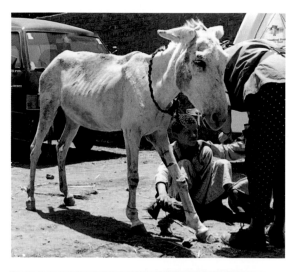

AUTHOR'S NOTE

It has been estimated that, annually, 20% of horses experience weight loss and 10% have diarrhoea as a result of worm damage. About 80% of colics are said to be related to worm problems.

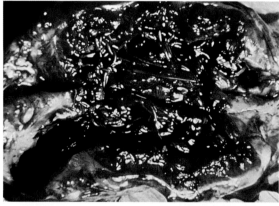

Parasites cause symptoms including
- Colic; severe, often fatal from physical obstruction in the gut, bowel damage preventing complete digestion or clots in the arteries to the intestine. The photo on the right shows large redworm in an artery.
- Loss of condition, weakness and lethargy
- Diarrhoea and dehydration
- Dull coat and pot-bellied appearance
- Loss of appetite
- Anaemia apparent from pale mucous membranes.
- Filled legs, abdomen and sheath
- Respiratory difficulties.

Eggs laid under the tail cause
- Intense itching. Worms as well as lice or sweet itch can cause tail rubbing, *see right*.

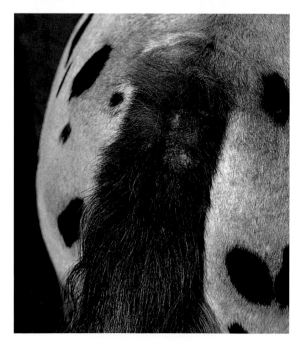

There may be worms visible in the dung
- Adult pinworms, tapeworms, large roundworms and small redworm larvae may be seen.

Often only some horses on the same grazing succumb to clinical disease at any one time. The weaker horses may have been forced to eat the poorer, larvae-infested grass and so have higher burdens. Also some horses seem to be genetically more prone to accumulating parasites. Look out for condition loss in only some members of the herd. If any symptoms are noticed, a vet should be consulted immediately. Symptoms can occur in different combinations and different degrees of severity, or may indicate other disorders.

Small Redworm Disease (*larval cyathostomosis*)   This is currently the most common problem associated with worms. Small redworm can be 90% of the worm burden and some of the 40 species which can infect horses have been shown to be resistant to Benzimidazole drugs. They have a short life cycle which enables rapid reproduction and they also encyst or 'hibernate' in the gut wall for periods of up to two years, so it is very difficult to clear a horse of worms. To understand why they cause such a problem, we need to return to the concept of overlap-

ping life cycles. In the summer the life cycle flows smoothly with steady numbers of larvae encysting and then emerging. The resulting damage can be repaired. In the autumn larvae stop emerging but are still being consumed and thus encysting. By springtime, there are huge numbers of encysted larvae. They then emerge simultaneously. The damage may be irreparable and can prove fatal within days. It is thought that a mass emergence can also occur up to two weeks after a heavily infested horse is wormed with a drug which only kills adult worms, so causing larvae to emerge to fill the gap. Symptoms include gradual or sudden weight loss, diarrhoea, colic and filled legs. Chances of survival are only 50%. Horses under six and over 15 are particularly vulnerable.

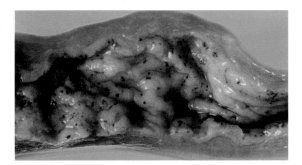

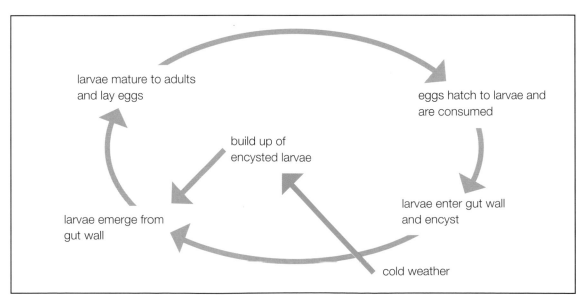

larvae mature to adults and lay eggs

eggs hatch to larvae and are consumed

build up of encysted larvae

larvae enter gut wall and encyst

larvae emerge from gut wall

cold weather

PASTURE MANAGEMENT

It has been shown that correct pasture management on its own can keep infection levels in the horse lower than drug treatment alone. Drugs have limited powers and are used routinely in horses to prevent build up of pasture contamination, not to treat disease. If a horse is already on contaminated pasture, immediately after being wormed he will ingest thousands more larvae which will damage him, complete their lifecycle and increase pasture contamination until the next dose. Correct pasture management ensures minimal infestation in the first place and drugs should be used to reduce that further. If drugs are used on their own, resistance to them will develop more easily, and a legacy of parasite resistance to all drugs may result for horses in the future. With careful pasture management, feed bills can be reduced and worming intervals can be taken to the maximum for each drug.

Why horses eat contaminated grass
- If a horse is lower down the pecking order he will be forced onto poorer, parasite-infested grass.
- If the whole field is rank, horses will eat what is available, from the rank contaminated grass to poisonous plants.

REDUCING CONTAMINATION

If the standard advice of removing dung twice weekly is not followed, it is likely you will have a badly contaminated field. It takes months, even years, to reduce contamination, but only weeks to create it. Many horse owners have limited grazing so there is not sufficient land to which horses may be moved while the fields are treated and rested. This can be disastrous. No matter how little space there is, there must be at least two separate areas in order to attempt correct pasture management.

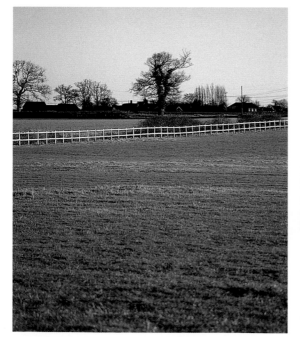

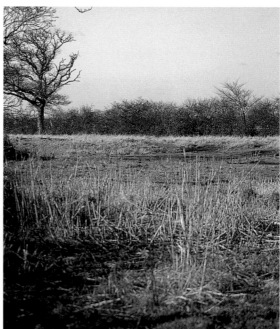

Divide the field into two equal sections with an electric fence. Ensure there is shelter, a gate and water on each side. This may take a while to organise, so immediately begin the removal of droppings.

Decide where to put the muck. A corner of the field is fine but in the long term it will need to be fenced. Local gardeners might be happy to take it away or, alternatively, put it on a trailer to be towed away.

In heavily soiled areas rake the dung into lines, then into heaps and finally onto an old blanket. Gather the corners together and drag the blanket away. This method avoids back strain. Since the area is contaminated anyway, raking will not spread larvae onto unsoiled areas.

Invest in a 'poop scoop' to clear the areas where dung piles are spread out and raking would contaminate clean ground. Again, tip the dung onto a blanket or use a wheelbarrow. Lifting dung with rubber gloves is tiring, making an unpleasant job even worse so it is unlikely to be done as regularly as it should. In winter, frozen manure is easier to lift with a broad shovel.

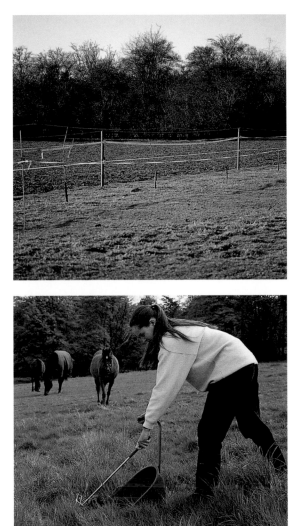

From now on, manure must be removed twice weekly before the eggs hatch, or once a week over the winter.

Once the field has been divided, the horses must be put onto a proper worming programme (see p.17).

Always worm horses the day they are moved onto rested land and pick up the droppings daily for three days. The drugs take a while to pass through the body and kill adults and eggs, so the horse will continue to pass viable eggs for a few days.

However, if the owner is scrupulous about removing the droppings, the eggs will not have time to hatch.

Contrary to popular belief, there is little point in worming horses a few days before leaving the old pasture as they may continue to pick up large numbers of larvae.

Rest the other half of the land for at least six weeks, ideally for four months, although this may not be practical if land is limited. This resting will partially reduce the pasture larval count.

Once the grass has benefited from the resting and has a stronger base and higher yield, each area can be rested for longer periods of time.

Try to find more land, so periodically each field can be rested for 4–6 months, without the field that is being used being grazed beyond recovery.

Grazing two cows or five sheep per acre on a field is good for growth and will further reduce contamination since equine parasites are destroyed inside cattle and sheep and the only parasite common to them all (stomach hairworm) is fairly easily controlled by routine worming. Remember the fencing will need to be

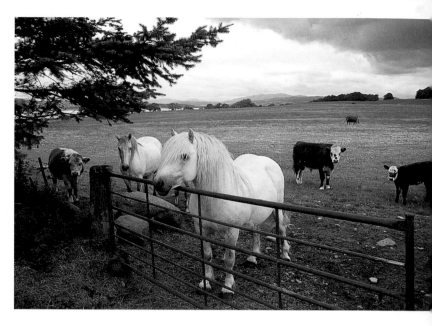

strong enough for sheep and cattle as well as being safe for horses.

Wet fields provide ideal conditions for parasites, and poor conditions for horses, so proper drainage may need to be considered.

USING MACHINERY

Suction cleaners are a valuable asset for larger establishments. They are fairly expensive – £2,000 upwards – but require little maintenance except regular cleaning. As well as removing manure from fields, they vacuum up leaves, grass, and hedge cuttings. For those who do not want a large outlay, cleaners may be hired. Suppliers advertise in equestrian magazines.

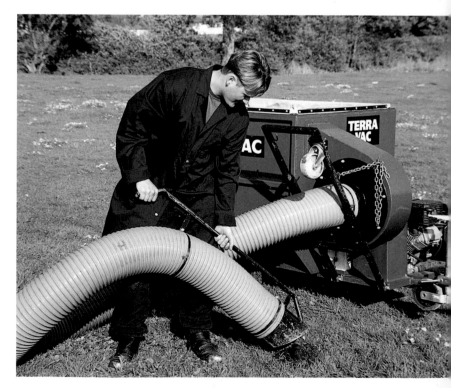

Harrowing prepares the ground for fertiliser and aerates the soil, promoting good growth. Traditionally, it has also been used to break up dung, exposing eggs and larvae to the sun to dry out and die. However, it has been shown that horses grazing on harrowed fields where dung has been spread in wet weather may have higher worm burdens than those where the dung is left. If eggs and larvae are spread over the grass and survive, horses cannot avoid them. Eggs can survive for months even when exposed. Some will be killed after four consecutive dry weeks at over 20 °C, allowing the horses to be put back soon after harrowing, but in the British climate, there is only a short period in the summer when this is possible. When fields are harrowed prior to fertilising in spring and autumn, the dung should ideally be removed first. If the horses have not

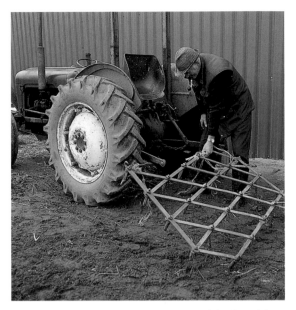

been wormed regularly, their fields should never be harrowed to spread dung unless the land can subsequently be rested for nine months.

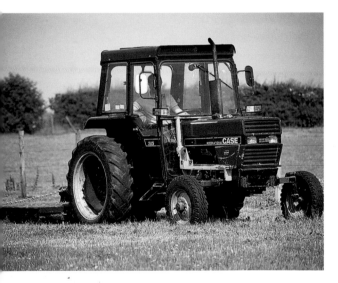

Topping does little, if anything, to reduce the larvae count. After cutting down grass with larvae at the top, the larvae still remain in the grass. However, topping is essential to promote even grass growth, and the subsequent resting of the fields will help to reduce the larvae count.

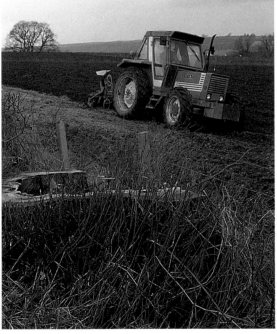

Ploughing is an option for an extremely horse-sick field and will dramatically reduce contamination.

PASTURE MANAGEMENT AT STUDS

Studs are very vulnerable to parasite problems as horses with unknown backgrounds regularly come on to the premises. Young horses are particularly susceptible to damage from all worms, particularly threadworm and large roundworm which only affect youngsters.

As can be seen from the photographs (comparison of large roundworm egg [above] and pinworm egg [below]), large roundworms cause problems because the eggs have a much thicker coating than other eggs so they can survive for years. For this reason, it would be wise for establishments with young horses to remove dung prior to harrowing for other reasons. Eggs can stick to the mare's udder and to the stable, so they must be cleaned regularly. Large roundworms grow quickly and within

a few weeks could cause an impaction. It is essential to minimise the number of larvae ingested by the foal.

A foal born early in the year and spending its first weeks inside can suffer catastrophic illness if turned onto even mildly contaminated land which other foals born at grass seem to tolerate. These foals need to be turned onto very clean pasture otherwise, if they do not gradually acquire a small infestation from the odd mouthful of grass over the first weeks, the sudden shock of infection by thousands of larvae can be too much.

Rotation of fields is crucial. A system like the leader-follower system should be used to ensure that foals never graze the same areas as foals from the previous year and that there is a rest period before foals graze an area recently grazed by adults. A stud must have a minimum of four areas which are rotated annually and subdivided to allow periodic resting during the year. Below is the plan for one area.

1st year:	3 months – cattle and sheep	
	9 months rest	
2nd year:	mares and foals	
3rd year:	youngsters	
4th year:	mature horses	

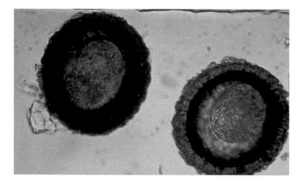

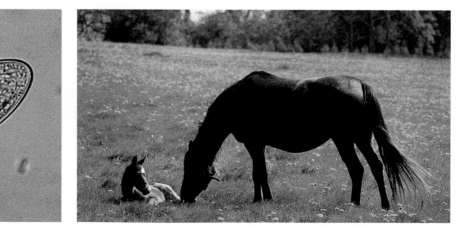

WORMING PROGRAMMES

Profile of drugs Worming drugs are also known as anthelmintics (anti-helminth) and can be purchased from vets, veterinary pharmacies, mail order companies or equestrian suppliers. Pharmacists must demonstrate 'due care and attention' when selling drugs and saddlers must ensure that the purchaser is a bona fide horse owner or keeper. If you are under 18 it may save embarrassment if you take an adult with you. Drugs should be stored in a cool, dry, locked cupboard away from children and other animals. Below are some of the most common drugs used.

Drugs and brand names	How they work	Frequency of dosing and contraindications	Worms they are effective against
Avermectin Group **Ivermectin** – *Eqvalan and Furexel.* Both are exactly the same drug in different packaging. Only available as a paste.	Paralysis and death of worms due to interference with the transmission of nerve impulses. Non-spastic paralysis.	8–10 weeks. If horse has large burdens of immature neck threadworm, there may be swelling and itching. It is not serious but if it persists call vet.	**Routine dose:** *Immature and adult* large redworm, small redworm, pinworm, large roundworm, lung-worm, *adult* threadworm, stomach worm, *immature* neck threadworm, *all stages* of bots.
Pyrimidine Group **Pyrantel Embonate** – *Pyratape P* and *Strongid P.* Both are exactly the same. The former is available in paste only. The latter in paste and granules.	Spastic paralysis of worms. Acts in gut, not in rest of body so only kills adult worms and eggs.	4–6 weeks. Not to be given to severely debilitated animals. Impaction of small intestine may occur in youngsters with significant numbers of large roundworm.	**Routine dose:** *adult* large redworm, small redworm, pinworm and large roundworm. **Double dose:** *adult* tapeworm.
Benzimidazole Group **Fenbendazole** – *Panacur.* Paste and granules.	Prevents uptake of food by worms.	6–8 weeks.	**Routine dose:** *adult* large redworm, small redworm (if no resistance), *immature and adult* pinworm and large roundworm.
Panacur Equine Guard Same as *Panacur*, but is standard dose given daily for five consecutive days. Available as a liquid.	Prevents uptake of food by worms.	Once or twice a year to complement a proper worming programme.	As above, but kills *adult* threadworm, and *immature* large redworm and small redworm and *encysted* small redworm.
Menbendazole – *Telmin.* Paste and granules.	Prevents uptake of food by worms.	Every 6 weeks.	**Routine dose:** *adult* large redworm, small redworm (if no resistance), large roundworm, pinworm, lungworm.
Oxibendazole – *Lincoln, Equitac, Equidin.* Paste.	Prevents uptake of food by worms.	6–8 weeks.	**Routine dose:** *adult* large redworm, small redworm (if no resistance), large roundworm, pinworm. **1.5 dose:** *adult* threadworm.

BASIC RULES

- All horses on the premises should be wormed with the same drug at the same time.
- If horses are being moved to clean pasture, worm them that day and pick up droppings daily for three days.
- Isolate new horses to the premises and after a few days use the worming programme (right), even if the horses were wormed fairly recently.
- For your own benefit, keep accurate records and retain receipts. Also, if you sell your horse you can prove he has been well looked after.

The sample worming programmes in this section are given as guidelines only.

Discuss the needs of your horse with your vet.

Worming an ill horse A horse which is very thin, showing symptoms of a worm problem, suffering from another illness, or is receiving medication should only be wormed following consultation with a vet.

Worming an apparently healthy horse which may have a large worm burden
Horses which fall into this category include any new horses to the premises (always assume they have a large burden) and horses which have never been wormed or have been wormed infrequently because their owners did not realise what was involved. The initial treatment programme should include drug groups which will remove all important worms. There are two additional points to bear in mind.

- A horse under two years old may have huge numbers of large roundworm. If these are killed all at once, especially by a drug which causes spastic paralysis as opposed to a non-spastic paralysis, they could cause an impaction. Fortunately this is fairly rare.
- All horses could have a massive burden of small redworm. If only the adult worms are removed, it could trigger a mass emergence of the remaining encysted larvae.

The programme below takes this into consideration.

Days 1–5: worm with *Panacur Equine Guard*, which is a five-day course of treatment. It is claimed that it gradually removes all stages of small redworm larvae and other worms.
Day 6: give a double dose of *Pyratape P* or *Strongid P* for tapeworm.
Week 4: dose with *Eqvalan* or *Furexel*, which will remove most remaining worms and in winter will remove bots.
Watch for any signs of colic over this period.
Then put onto the same preventative programme as other horses.

AUTHOR'S NOTE

It has been estimated that two out of three DIY livery yards do not have a proper worming programme. If your horse is at one of these yards, insist a proper programme is started now.

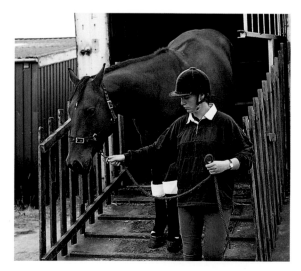

STANDARD PREVENTATIVE PROGRAMMES

Horses on very clean grazing because of ample acreage and/or scrupulous hygiene, or those which are stabled and turned out onto clean grazing, can be wormed at the maximum interval given for each drug. Horses which are on horse-sick or overcrowded grazing, even for a few hours a day, should be wormed at the minimum intervals.

This situation must be remedied as soon as possible. There are certain times of year when particular parasites need to be targeted by certain drugs. The drugs used at other times can be rotated annually among Ivermectin, Pyrantel and also Benzimidazoles if there is no resistance.

Month	Clean Grazing Year 1	Poor Grazing Year 1	Clean Grazing Year 2	Poor Grazing Year 2	Clean Grazing Year 3	Poor Grazing Year 3
Mid January						
End January						
Mid February						
End February		Ivermectin		Pyrantel		Benzimidazole
Mid March	Ivermectin		Pyrantel		Benzimidazole	
End March				Pyrantel		
Mid April						Benzimidazole
End April		Ivermectin	Pyrantel	Pyrantel		
Mid May					Benzimidazole	
End May	Ivermectin			Pyrantel		Benzimidazole
Mid June			Pyrantel			
End June		Ivermectin		Pyrantel		
Mid July					Benzimidazole	Benzimidazole
End July			Pyrantel	Pyrantel		
Mid August	Ivermectin					
End August		Ivermectin		Pyrantel		Benzimidazole
Mid Sept			Pyrantel		Benzimidazole	
End Sept						
Mid October	Double dose Pyrantel – tapeworm					
End October						
Mid November	5 day Fenbendazole – encysted redworm					
End November						
Mid December						
End December	Ivermectin – bot larvae					

EXCEPTIONS TO THE RULE

Horses with resistant worms If, after dung analysis, it appears that Benzimidazole drugs are not effective, alternate between the sample programmes given for year 1 and year 2. Still use the five-day dose of Fenbendazole as at this level it is claimed to kill most resistant worms.

Old horses Add a five-day dose of Fenbendazole at the beginning of February.

Horses which have recovered from clinical worm disease Put onto clean grazing and start with the first year programme. Add another five-day dose of Fenbendazole in February.

Pregnant mares Worm as normal throughout pregnancy except where unusual drugs give warnings otherwise. Worm with Ivermectin within 24 hours after foaling to prevent transfer of threadworms to foal in milk. Unless willing to do regular worm counts, studs should assume Benzimidazole resistance in the small redworms and alternate between years 1 and 2 of programme.

Foals If a foal has diarrhoea, call a vet. If it is confirmed to be due to threadworm, the vet will advise on treatment. On studs where there is a problem, foals can be wormed at two weeks under veterinary supervision. Otherwise start worming at four to six weeks and every eight weeks thereafter, at the same time as the dam. Use Ivermectin which at routine dose kills all worms which are a threat to foals. From six months, integrate into normal programme.

Donkeys Donkeys are affected by the same worms as horses. Although donkeys are the natural host to lungworm, it is perfectly safe to mix donkeys and horses

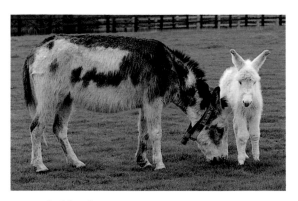

provided both are on proper worming programmes. Ivermectin is effective against larval and adult lungworm, so should be used regularly. Alternate between year 1 and either year 2 or year 3 programme (if no resistance). The Donkey Sanctuary worms new donkeys with Ivermectin approximately one week after arrival and four to six weeks later before leaving isolation. Donkeys weigh 165–185 kg, so one syringe of Ivermectin will give three treatments. Old or sick donkeys should only be wormed following consultation with a vet.

ADMINISTRATION OF DRUGS

Before administering any drugs, it is necessary to establish the weight of the horse. Weight can be calculated by using a weighbridge, a special weighband which estimates the weight by the girth measurement, or by

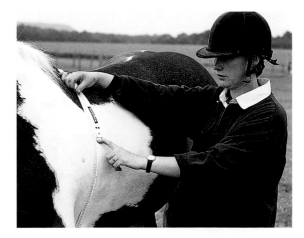

using the formula below. There is no need to starve a horse before dosing with modern wormers.

$$\frac{\text{Girth (cm)} \times \text{Length (cm)}}{8717} = \text{Weight (kg)}$$

Length is from point of shoulder to point of buttock.

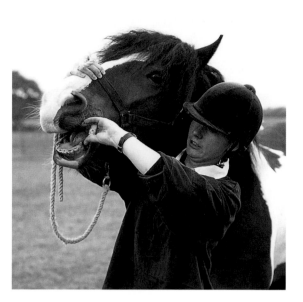

AUTHOR'S NOTE

Safety Always have the horse untied and wear a hat if he is awkward. If in a stable, ensure it has a high roof. Ask an assistant to help if necessary.

Syringe

- Unfortunately, syringes are usually white – the worst colour to have close to a headshy horse! Always adjust the syringe out of sight of the horse and have it ready in your pocket. Check his mouth is empty as it is easier for him to spit out the paste if it is coating food.

- Firmly insert the syringe in the interdental space and aim it towards the back of the mouth. Quickly squirt it onto the tongue. When withdrawing the syringe, roll it on the tongue to remove any paste still sticking to it.

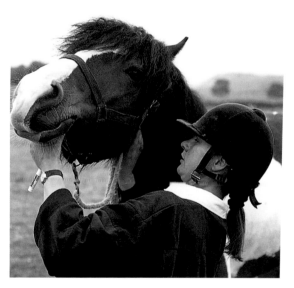

- Lift the horse's head up until he has swallowed and prevent him from eating for the next few minutes.

- Always have another syringe on standby. If any paste is dropped, the dose can be topped up, so it is not all wasted.

Awkward horses It is sometimes easier to hold the underneath of the headcollar noseband than putting your arm under and

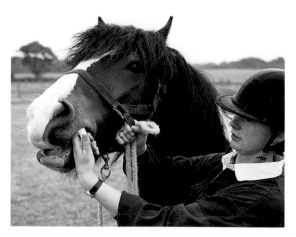

round the horse's nose. Alternatively, try threading the leadrope through the offside ring of the noseband, over the nose and then through the nearside ring. If the horse throws his head up, the downward pressure should give more control. Ideally an assistant should be on hand to hold an awkward horse.

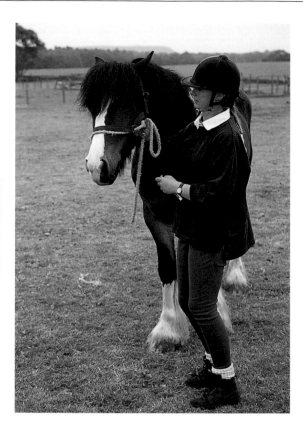

> **AUTHOR'S NOTE**
>
> Some wormers only come in a syringe but the paste can be mixed in the feed if it is less trouble.

In the feed The problem with this method is that if the feed is not eaten all at once, the drug may not reach the required concentration in the body to kill the worms. Fortunately most granules are palatable. Usually the drug would be mixed with a smaller feed given at the usual time. With difficult characters, some owners give a small feed and then half an hour later give another small feed with the drug added. If that does not work, adding molasses to the feed can disguise the different taste. Remember to keep the feed small so that it is all eaten.

> **AUTHOR'S NOTE**
>
> When giving drugs, the feed must always be in a container, not fed straight from the ground. Ensure no horse can eat a dose intended for another.

Panacur Equine Guard is a liquid which is mixed into the feed. It is possible to draw small amounts into a plastic syringe to administer it but it does not stick to the tongue like a paste and can run out more easily.

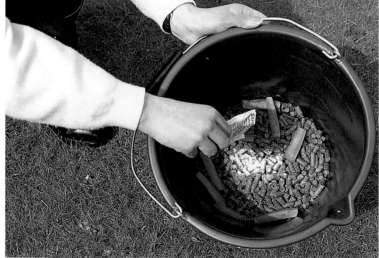

If you cannot get drugs of any sort into your horse, ask your vet for advice.

TESTS TO HELP WITH A WORMING PROGRAMME

FAECAL EGG COUNT

Analysis of manure is the obvious starting point when estimating the extent of a worm burden. It usually costs less than a dose of wormer to have a sample analysed. The owner provides the vet with a small sample of fresh dung. If it is estimated that there are more than 100–200 eggs per gram of manure then undesirable levels of parasites are present. This proce-

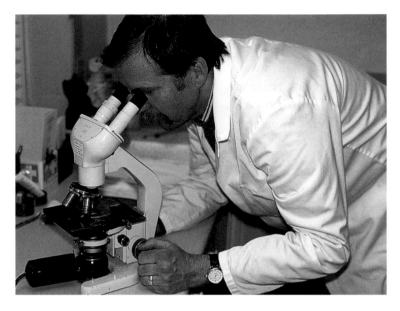

dure is often used to check if a worming programme is working. All horses on overcrowded grazing should be tested twice a year. Large establishments may choose to check a sample of horses. All horses wormed with Benzimidazole drugs should be tested in spring and autumn. If a dung sample is analysed just before worming and another a few days after, the reduction in the number of eggs should be more than 70%. If not, there could be a problem with parasite resistance.

When a very low egg count is found before worming, it is tempting to discontinue the worming programme but the result has shown that the programme is correct and should therefore be maintained, although drugs could be extended to their maximum intervals. It is possible to do egg counts every month from spring to autumn and only use drugs when the count is more than 100–200 per gram, but it may be more expensive than following a standard drug programme. It would only be economic

for the owner with few horses on a substantial acreage.

There are limitations with faecal egg counts.
• In winter when huge numbers of small redworm are encysted they will not lay eggs, so an egg count at this time would not reflect the extent of the problem.
• Lungworm and liverfluke may never reach the egg laying stage in the horse but are still present and causing damage.
• Egg counts can vary from day to day.

BLOOD TESTING

Clinical signs of worm problems are often non-specific so blood analysis can assist diagnosis. In equines, eosinophil counts are normally 2% and can rise to 6–8% in infested animals. The average owner will not use blood testing as part of a worm prevention programme but competition horses may have regular blood analysis so any problems such as a worm burden can be dealt with before they affect performance.

OTHER WAYS OF BREAKING LIFE CYCLES

Although good pasture management and use of drugs are the main ways to break life cycles, there are some extra steps which can be taken for specific parasites.

• From July to September in the southern two thirds of the country, check neck, legs and belly daily for bot eggs and remove with a grooming block or bot knife in the direction of hair growth. Apply fly repellents and ensure no horse grazes alone – horses protect each other from flies.

• Pinworms lay eggs under the horse's tail so use a separate sponge for the dock area.

• In a stable, eggs can adhere to walls and fixtures. All containers must be cleaned regularly and the stable steam cleaned or disinfected from time to time. Steam cleaning is more effective against large roundworm eggs, so could be used in establishments with young horses.

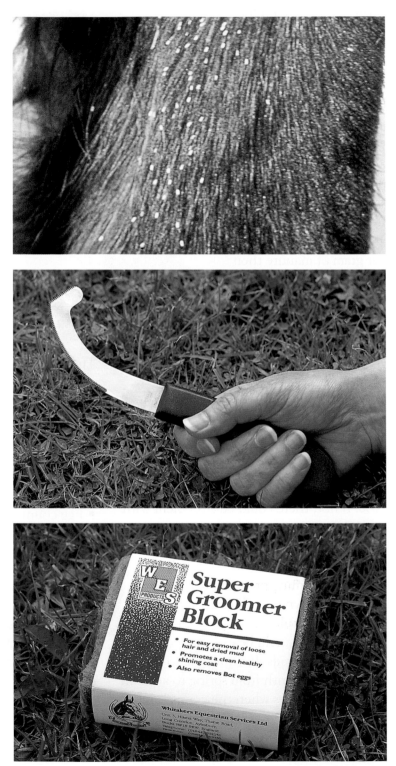

CONCLUSION

It may be tempting after reading the horror story of parasites to think that the easiest way to prevent the problem is to stable the horse 24 hours a day, isolated from others. Of course, in clinical terms this will reduce the ingestion of parasites but would be cruel to the horse. We must give him as much space as possible to graze, exercise and enjoy the company of other equines. We have created the parasite problem by restricting the horse. In the wild a horse would rarely accumulate numbers sufficient to cause trouble. It is our duty to manage the problem so the horse can still enjoy a little of what is natural to him. It may seem to be a lot of effort to muck out our fields and expensive to buy drugs but in the end it is economical – prevention being better than the cure.

I hope I have dispelled the myth that donkeys and horses cannot graze together because of lungworm. It is tragic to think of a donkey or horse being denied company merely because their owner did not understand how easy it was, with the correct use of drugs and pasture management, to prevent a parasite problem.

NEW DEVELOPMENTS AND RESEARCH

Statistics gathered during a recent epidemiological study have suggested a small possibility of a link between regular worming and an increased risk of grass sickness. At the time of writing, the opinion of those who conducted the study is that this information should have no impact on current worming programmes, unless future research changes this view.

Drugs must go through rigorous testing to be licensed and must be licensed before they can be called wormers. The cost of this research and licensing means that we will see few, if any, new drug groups developed. Moxidectin from the Avermectin drug group may be available from 1999. It can be used as an alternative to Ivermectin, although the dosing intervals may be different. There is hope that in future decades a vaccine may be developed to help a horse acquire immunity to parasites. Recently homeopathic worm remedies have appeared on the market but owners should be aware that they are not licensed wormers and there is only anecdotal evidence as to their efficacy. If, in the future, they are proven to be effective, they could be a valuable alternative to conventional drugs. In the meantime, if tempted to use them, owners would be wise to consult a vet and have regular egg counts done.

CHECKLIST

To break life cycles in as many ways as possible:

- Fields should have dung removed twice weekly, be rested regularly, be rotated with cattle and sheep and have good drainage.
- When moved to clean land, horses should be wormed and droppings removed daily for three days.
- All new horses to a yard should be wormed appropriately.
- All horses should be wormed at the same time with the same drug.
- Fly repellents should be used in areas where bots are present.
- Bot eggs must be removed.
- Stables should be steam cleaned or disinfected regularly.

ACKNOWLEDGEMENTS

I should like to express my thanks to all those who helped me in the preparation of this book: Andrew Trawford, BVSc, MSc, of The Donkey Sanctuary; Deborah Baker, BVet Med, MRCVS, of Hoechst (UK) Ltd and James Wood of the Animal Health Trust for supplying useful information; Sue Gooding of The Donkey Sanctuary, and Sue Tilly of Terra Vac for providing photographs; Deborah Murray and Andrew Couper of Westmuir Riding Centre, West Lothian, George MacRitchie, BVMS, MRCVS, Drum Feeds, Danderhall, Edinburgh, Ian and Elizabeth Comrie, Houston Farm Riding School, Uphall, West Lothian and George Millar for assisting with location photographs. My special thanks go to Derek Braid for all his time and effort, to Jane Parry, BVet Med, MRCVS of MERIEL who provided all the laboratory photographs together with much useful information, to Professor James Duncan, BVMS, PhD, MRCVS of the Department of Veterinary Medicine, University of Glasgow for his useful comments on my manuscript and to my parents who encouraged and supported me when worms threatened to take over my life.

Photographic Acknowledgements:
MERIEL, Sandringham House, Harlow Business Park, Harlow, Essex, CM19 5TG; Terra Vac, a division of Vulcan Engineers Ltd., Unit 2, Melbourne Bridge, Haverhill, Suffolk, CB9 7RR. 01440 712171; The Donkey Sanctuary, Sidmouth, Devon, EX10 0NU; Jane van Lennep; all other photographs, Derek Braid.

British Library Cataloguing-in-Publication Data.
A catalogue record for this book is available from the
British Library

ISBN 0.85131.709.X

First published in Great Britain 1999 by
J.A.Allen
Clerkenwell House
Clerkenwell Green
London EC1R 0HT

J.A.Allen is an imprint of Robert Hale Limited

Design and Typesetting by Paul Saunders
Series editor Jane Lake
Printed in Hong Kong by Midas Printing International Ltd.